GW01036321

GUT BALANCE SOLUTION

10 steps on how you can restore optimal gut health, boost metabolism and heal your gut effectively

By GERARD JOHNSON

TABLE OF CONTENT

Avocado and Spinach Shake

FOR SNACKS AND SALADS, YOU CAN TRY THESE
GUT-BALANCE DRESSINGS AND DIPS

Avocado Dressing

Best Balsamic Dressing

Gut-Balance Caesar Dressing

Ginger Dressing

Guacamole Dip

Zucchini Hummus

Sunflower Seed Pate

For LUNCH AND DINNER, here are our TOP 8 choices:

Chicken Nuggets with Thai Dipping Sauce

Summer Vegetable Kelp Noodles

Spaghetti Squash with Cauliflower Sauce

Parchment Halibut with Olives

Thai Coconut Chicken Soup

Gingered Salmon Stir Fry

Coriander Crusted Halibut

Summer Squash and Tomato Bake

Conclusion

Legal & Disclaimer

Legal & Disclaimer

professional medical advice before using any of the suggested remedies, techniques, or information in this book.

Upon using the information contained in this book, you agree to hold harmless the Author from and against any damages, costs, and expenses, including any legal fees potentially resulting from the application of any of the information provided by this guide. This disclaimer applies to any damages or injury caused by the use and application, whether directly or indirectly, of any advice or information presented, whether for breach of contract, tort, negligence, personal injury, criminal intent, or under any other cause of action.

Introduction

The state of your gut says a lot about you. By taking time to know how healthy your digestive track is, you'll get a good idea of how good your overall health is. If your gut is leaky or you are suffering from a bowel disorder, there's a good chance that you're affected by other mental and autoimmune disorders as well. A poor gut health, particularly if there are more bad bacteria than good, can also affect the way you feel. It can trigger mood changes- making you feel more irritable and grumpy.

Aside from emotions and mood, an imbalance in your digestive track, specifically serotonin circulation, can also lead to mental health issues. Serotonin is a brain neurotransmitter that works to regulate mood and appetite. It also plays a vital role in a person's memory and learning. Around 90% of our serotonin supply comes from our digestive track. If this serotonin supply becomes insufficient, cognitive function gets impaired and risks for mental problems, like Parkinson's disease, increase greatly.

Knowing how your gut health can predispose you to several illnesses can be alarming. Fortunately, there's something you can do about it and *you can start with this book now.*

Gut healing is not an overnight process. Instead, it takes time, commitment and effort on your part to make the necessary adjustments possible. Generally speaking, there are four main steps that you need to follow in order to achieve optimum gut health. This involves the processes of Removal, Replacement, Re-inoculation and Repair. These steps seem easy at first glance; however, because they involve lifestyle change, they can be challenging for most people.

This book has broken down those steps into specific details which you can easily incorporate to your daily living. They are simple to follow but are guaranteed to help improve your gut, heal your digestive system and prevent debilitating and annoying illnesses from happening to you.

Gut health is crucial to your well-being. As the Father of Modern Medicine, Hippocrates, once said, "All disease begins in the gut".

Chapter 1

Why Gut Health is Important

The gut, or the gastrointestinal track, plays a crucial role in your overall health. It is responsible for 70% of your immunity. It's the largest endocrine organ in the body and it acts as your second brain. It produces vitamins, excretes waste products and keeps your hormones in check.

Apparently, that's not all there is to your gut.

Several studies have also linked the digestive track with various aspects of the human health. One of these notable links involves the presence of the millions of bacteria in your gut and your capability to protect yourself against diseases. When your gut has more bad bacteria than the good ones, your body's ability to detoxify harmful substances and eliminate them from your system decreases. In contrast, when you have more good bacteria, your body will be more resistant against diseases.

The environment of your intestinal track also plays a major role in keeping toxins from entering your blood stream. The cellular lining as well as its chemical barriers protects your body from possible pathogens. Any alteration to these components predisposes you to cases such as cancer, depression and even obesity.

Weakening and the increased permeability of the intestinal walls, also known as leaky gut syndrome, can trigger several health issues. Because the walls are more permeable, toxins and waste products leak out and trigger an immune system reaction. It can cause food allergies, arthritis, autism and even learning difficulties.

Aside from your immunity, your gut also plays a major role in your mental health. In fact, your gut has its own nervous system that shoots information to your brain. This is more commonly known as your enteric nervous system and it's responsible for the upset stomach you experience when you're angry or when you're tensed. It's also the reason why you feel butterflies in your stomach when you're nervous.

The link between your gut and your brain causes mental issues like anxiety and depression. Serotonin specifically plays a major role in why these mental conditions happen in a person. Serotonin is a neurotransmitter that is involved in several brain functions. It affects your mood, sleep and appetite. Although it is more associated with mental functions, a large percentage of serotonin is concentrated and produced in your gut. If the body's requirement for this neurotransmitter is not met or if you're gut is not healthy enough to produce serotonin, your mental health can suffer.

Our digestive track is responsible for what we eat and what we excrete. If it fails to break down the food we put inside our mouth, we will not be able to receive the nutrients we need for optimum health. On such note, if the gut fails to eliminate toxins and they accumulate inside the body, the system becomes toxic and we become sick.

The importance of gut health is easy to understand. Making sure it stays on top shape, however, is a different and more complicated story. With all the unhealthy food choices and habits today, it's not surprising to find more people getting sick every day. If your health is currently suffering or you just want to be healthy, you can start repairing your health by listening to what your gut has to say. If your gut is healthy, so are you.

Chapter 2

Worst Foods for Your Gut

The first step in fixing your gut health is eliminating the factors that pose harm to it. Introducing healthy foods or incorporating a new health regime can't really help you in improving your gut health if won't delete the bad factors first. They will only negate and outdo all your efforts. When this happens, the process towards a healthier digestive system can get frustrating and you'll end up throwing your hands in the air.

To avoid this from happening, here's a list of the foods you should be taking out first:

Chlorinated Water

Water, on its own, is essential for your health. Chlorinated water, on the other hand, isn't. The added chlorine kills the bacteria in your water to make it safe to drink. The problem with chlorine, however, is it tends to kill all bacteria- both good and bad.

Your gut needs good bacteria to function effectively. These bacteria are important in maintaining the natural environment and processes of your digestive track. Without them, the processes of digestion, assimilation and vitamin production would be impaired. Similar to a domino effect, a change in the balance between the good and bad bacteria can trigger a lot of health issues. For one, your ability to ward off diseases will be lessened if the normal flora of your gut is altered. Your mood and ability to concentrate will also be affected. You'll be more prone to stomach ache, bloating and even inflammation of your gut.

Drinking chlorinated water can also nullify any effort you're doing at probiotic supplementation. Even if you're modifying your diet to introduce more good bacteria, the chlorine in your water will only eliminate them.

Spices

Excessively spicy foods aren't good for your gut. As they are actually a mixture of acids, consuming them greatly doubles the acid present in your stomach's environment. This results to several reactions.

Inflammation of the gastric lining is very common among people who eat spicy foods. Over time, inflammation turns to irritation and the gastric wall becomes weakened. On severe cases, spicy foods lead to the ulceration of the walls of the stomach, duodenum and even the esophagus. One person can develop multiple ulcers in varying parts of his gut. These ulcers are painful and can cause great discomfort. If they are triggered, ulcers can bleed. This bleeding is usually evident in a person's stool or vomit.

Acid reflux can also develop in people who consume too many spices. This happens when the muscular valve of the esophagus becomes weak. The excessive acid, without an effective valve, can travel upwards to the esophagus. Because the esophageal area is not used to being exposed to acid, a reflux can cause irritation and erosion of the esophageal lining.

Spicy foods can also cause excessive discomfort in people who have existing hemorrhoids. Although spices don't directly cause hemorrhoids to develop, their acidic nature further irritates and aggravates the condition.

Fatty Foods

Fatty foods are considered double edged when it comes to gut health. They can either slow down or speed up your metabolism and can result to either diarrhea or constipation. Aside from this, foods high in saturated fat are also more difficult to digest than other food types. Because they are harder to digest, the tendency of your stomach is to produce more acid in an attempt to break them easier.

The problem, however, occurs when there's too much acid in your stomach. Primarily, there's the risk of inflammation and irritation of your gastric lining. Also, when there's too much pressure, the valve on your esophagus may not be able to contain down the acid. As a result, reflux happens.

Fatty foods also have the ability to alter the normal flora in your gut. Because the microbes in your digestive track and your brain are strongly linked to each other, the resulting change equate to a disruption in how your brain normally functions.

Coffee

Coffee doesn't only wake you up. It also stimulates your gut to produce more acid to hasten food processing. When food processing goes faster than how it normally happens, food is transferred to the small intestine without getting fully digested. As a result, the undigested food remains in the small gut for a long time and associated toxicity results.

Coffee can also trigger inflammation response in the gut. Certain components of coffee cause bloating, cramping and increased peristalsis. Thus, it intensifies the symptoms of people with Irritable Bowel Syndrome and colitis. Heartburn is another a common condition associated with regular drinkers of coffee. Acid reflux results from the inability of the valve in the esophagus to keep the acid down in the stomach. Acid, reaching areas of the digestive track where it isn't supposed to reach, can cause not only irritation but ulceration as well.

Gluten

Gluten is a type of protein that binds the nutrients you'll find in grains, such as wheat, barley and rye. Because of its binding property, most bread, when eaten, transforms into a sticky and pasty substance. Breaking gluten down into its building blocks is relatively easy for people without sensitivity to it. However, with people who are allergic to gluten, it's another more complicated story.

Gluten breakdown for people who are allergic to it involves an immune response. Their gut immunity finds gluten's building blocks as enemies which they have to eliminate. This immune response decreases their intestinal wall's ability to absorb nutrients and thus cause it to become leaky. Symptoms such as bloating, cramping and malnutrition subsequently follow.

Cold Foods

Internally, the human body is warm. This type of environment is important for homeostasis to happen. When you eat cold foods, this balance becomes disrupted. As form of compensation, your gut has to use great effort to warm these foods down to the right temperature.

Stress isn't the only harm done to the gut whenever you eat or drink something called. It also tends to render it inefficient in digesting. As a result, foods eaten cold are not thoroughly processed and indigestion, bloating as well as stomach pain develops.

People react differently. One person may react negatively to eggs while another person may not have any problems consuming it. This makes it important that you listen to what your body has to say. Be attentive to your body's reaction whenever you eat something new. If you need to eliminate foods in your diet, be sure to do it one by one. This will enable you to know exactly what reactions you get and from which food.

Chapter 3

Foods to Supercharge Your Gut

Improving your gut health doesn't stop at removing all the foods that can harm it. Actually, it's only the start of the process. Once you are able to take away all the bad foods in your kitchen, the next thing you should do is to replace them with healthier ones.

To enhance your gut, you need to replenish it with the essential nutrients and vitamins it needs to function at its best. One way you could do that is by eating foods that will supercharge your digestive track. Superfoods, on such note, can be your best solution.

Superfoods are packed with greater amounts of nutrients, vitamins and antioxidants than your regular fruits and vegetables. Because they are nutrient dense, these foods can do a lot for your body.

They can help prevent cancer, diabetes and several heart problems. Superfoods can also address various digestive health issues.

To help boost your gut health, you need to incorporate these foods in your daily diet:

Ghee

Ghee is a common cooking ingredient in the Southern parts of Asia. Technically, it is made of butter. However, unlike other butter byproducts, it undergoes prolonged cooking time to remove any solid ingredients and excess moisture. Because of this, ghee is more commonly referred to as "clarified butter". You can use it as a replacement to your regular cooking oil and butter.

Because it is a form of fat, consuming Ghee on a daily basis can help you absorb more of the fat soluble vitamin A, D, E and K. Ghee is also effective in addressing problems of indigestion by stimulating digestive enzyme production. These enzymes help hasten food processing in your gut. Aside from indigestion, ghee can assist in the healing of your digestive track as well. It lowers the production of stomach acid and aids in the repair of your gut lining.

It is also considered a potent anti-viral agent because of its rich butyric acid content.

Bone Broth

Bone broth is helpful among people with leaky gut syndrome. It contains a jelly like substance that works to seal the gut lining while facilitating its healing. Aside from leaky gut syndrome, bone broth is also effective in managing constipation. It attracts liquids inside your gut to make elimination easier.

Bone broth is also a source of Glycine. It helps increase the acid production in your stomach to help keep Irritable Bowel Syndrome and acid reflux at bay. Aside from Glycine, it also contains Glutamin which is considered as fuel for the cells in your small intestines. Since bones are made up of proteins, broths made out of bones are also rich sources of protein. Collagen and gelatin, which are forms of protein, are effective in managing ulceration in the gastric mucosa.

Kombucha

Kombucha, simply put, is a type of fermented tea. It is made out of sugar, tea and starter mushroom called

Scoby. Because of its benefit to the body, it has been widely used in several cultures and traditions.

Kombucha contains probiotics, enzymes and acids to assist in better digestion. It's also an effective detoxification agent. Aside from this, drinking Kombucha can also assist your gut in assimilating foods better to help avoid indigestion and several other gut problems.

Kefir

Kefir is somewhat similar with yogurt. The difference, however, lies in how they are made. Kefir contains yeast and bacteria and is made with grains that continuously multiply with each batch you create. Although it's a byproduct of milk, Kefir is safe to consume for people with lactose intolerance. The bacteria and yeast feed on the milk to render it lactose free.

Kefir does a lot for your body, particularly your gut. For one, it works as a probiotic supplement to enhance the good bacteria in your gut. Because it improves your gut's environment, Kefir is effective for people with leaky gut syndrome, Crohn's disease and

Irritable Bowel Syndrome. It also aids in faster metabolism to assist you in your weight loss goal.

Moringa

Moringa is a great source of fiber. It's often used in detoxification because of its ability to help get rid of the toxins inside the body. It also assists in the formation and proliferation of the good bacteria in your gut.

Aside from fiber, Moringa also has antibacterial properties. It contains Isothiocyanates that is considered effective in combating Helicobacter Pylori. H. Pylori is the main culprit in cases of gastritis, stomach and duodenal cancers.

Chapter 4

Eating Habits You Should Follow

Food choices aren't the only factors affecting your gut health. The way you eat and how much you eat also say a lot about how well your digestive track is. If you are a stress eater or you submit yourself to strict dieting, there's a good chance you could be harming your gut.

Never skip your breakfast. As much as it sounds like a cliché, eating the first meal of the day can do your gut health right. Aside from giving you the energy you'll need for your daily activities, eating breakfast can also help you steer away from unhealthy food choices. Additionally, breakfast prepares your metabolism for your subsequent meals. By warming up your metabolism, you're primarily stimulating it to work more efficiently. Failure to do so, on the other hand, can result to sluggish ability to metabolize foods, weight gain and bloating.

Chew your food properly. Breaking down food is already a tedious task for your gut. Improperly chewed foods, meanwhile, are far more strenuous for your digestion. Not only will your gut need to produce more acid, it will also be forced to work harder to break the pieces effectively. Gulping down food without chewing them properly can result to excessive gas and bloating.

Eat in moderate proportions. Eating too much food in a single meal serving can cause stomach pain and indigestion. Instead of having three large meals a day, you can choose to break your meals into six small sets. This way, it will be easier for your gut to process the food effectively and efficiently.

Avoid eating right away when you're stressed. Eating when stressed can cause bloating and indigestion. This results from the activation of your sympathetic nervous system in response to its perceived stress. When this system is triggered, your digestive system gets shut down to allow more blood and oxygen to reach the organs necessary for the fight or flight response. With less blood to the digestive track, the foods you introduce will not be effectively processed. Instead of working on your plate right away, take a few deep breaths to calm your system first. Deep breathing is considered effective in managing stress.

Drink enough water. Hydration is essential for your gut health. Drinking enough water every day can help make sure it functions at its best. Water serves as lubrication to your gut. When there is enough lubrication, peristalsis or the movement of food through your digestive track happens smoothly. Hydration, however, does not involve carbonated drinks and fruit juices. These drinks contain too much sugar that can serve as good food sources for the bad bacteria in your gut.

Listen to your gut. Loose bowel movements, cramping and bloating are signs that something is wrong with your gut. However, it doesn't readily mean that your digestive system is suffering from a disease. Most of the time, gut symptoms mean you're doing something wrong. By taking time to understand those symptoms and what their probable causes are, you'll get a good idea on how you'll be able to permanently avoid them.

Chapter 5

Essential Digestive Health Supplements

Most of the time, your body can't do healing on its own. This is particularly true in cases where damage has been extensive or your gut isn't strong enough to recover by itself. This makes supplementation necessary.

Deglycyrrhizinated Licorice

Licorice root has been a part of traditional medicine for several years already. It has both anti-inflammatory and antibacterial property. However, with prolonged use, licorice has been closely linked with cases of hypertension and other adverse reactions.

Deglycyrrhizinated licorice, or DGL, is created out of whole licorice but underwent further processing to remove Glycyrrhizin which largely contributes to elevated blood pressure. DGL, as a supplement, supports the proliferation of the mucus secreting cells of the gut and prolong gastric cellular life. It also improves the circulation in the gut and assist in its healing. DGL is effective to use in cases of peptic ulcers as well as Gastro-intestinal Reflux Disease.

Betaine Hydrochloric Acid

Low levels of stomach acid can lead to several problems. Primarily, an acidic environment is needed to make sure bad bacteria don't proliferate. Indigestion, acid reflux and nutrient deficiencies are also caused by insufficient acid in the stomach.

To compensate for this, you can supplement with Betaine Hydrochloric Acid. This supplement helps increase the acidity and amount of acid in your stomach. Although helpful with people who don't produce enough HCL in their gut, there are also people who need to skip this supplement. This includes people who are under corticosteroid therapy and those suffering from ulcers of the digestive track.

L-Glutamine

L-Glutamine is essentially a form of amino acid. It helps the body synthesize nucleic acid as well as protein. In terms of your gut health, L-Glutamine works to protect the mucosal lining of your digestive track. It also decreases the proliferation of bad bacteria while preventing natural cell death in the area.

Because of these properties, L-Glutamine is considered as effective in managing or even reversing the damages created by the leaky gut syndrome. Because the condition primarily affects the lining of the gut and its ability to serve as a barrier, you can rely on glutamine as support.

Slippery Elm

Slippery elm comes from the inner bark of the elm tree. It's widely used in parts of Northern America to relieve ailments, particularly of the digestive track. Slippery elm triggers natural mucus secretion. Mucus, as we all know, is important in that it coats and protects the lining of the gut. This mechanism helps greatly in avoiding ulcer formation as well as in preventing further damage to existing ulcers.

This supplement also aids in removing toxins inside your gut. It helps hasten food processing and the time it takes to transfer the food in the track. Aside from this, slippery elm also has the ability to add bulk and soften stool to facilitate easier elimination. It's equally effective in reducing inflammation and irritation in the gut caused by Irritable Bowel Syndrome and colitis.

Digestive Enzymes

Digestive enzymes naturally occur in your gut to help break down food into a form that it can easily absorb. If these enzymes become insufficient, such as with age or certain diseases, the gastrointestinal track becomes less efficient with its job. Not all digestive enzyme supplements are created equal. If you are new to purchasing this type of supplement, you should be looking out for one that has enzymes capable of helping you digest protein, fats and carbohydrates.

Aloe Vera

Aloe Vera is good for your skin. It's an effective moisturizer and a scar remover. Aside from these benefits, aloe Vera is also good for your digestive health. Primarily, it helps enhance digestion through its cleansing effect on the gut. This effect is not only limited to your stomach or your duodenum but the entire digestive track. Aloe Vera has an anti-inflammatory effect and can soothe ulcers and irritated gastric linings. If you are suffering from constipation, taking aloe Vera can help you as it is also considered an effective laxative.

Aloe Vera can be used fresh. It's actually the safer means of reaping the benefits of the plant. However, if you don't have immediate access to aloe Vera plant, you always have the option to buy from suppliers. If you are taking it in supplement form, take time and exercise caution in studying the brand and the supplement. You should also be aware of how much and how long you're allowed to take aloe Vera supplements. Most of the time, your attending health care specialist can give you an exact duration.

Chapter 6

Smoking Cessation and Your Digestive Health

Smoking can do a lot of damage to your gut. For one, it decreases the amount of mucus produced by the lining of your digestive track. This greatly decreases your gut's protection against ulceration and injury. Other than mucus, smoking can also lead to a decreased blood flow in your gut. If there isn't enough blood circulating around the area, healing as well as your gut's normal processes will be impaired.

Acid reflux is also commonly associated with people who frequently smoke. This usually happens as a result of the weakening of the lower esophageal sphincter. LES is a muscular valve that keeps the stomach's content from travelling upwards to the esophagus. Acid reflux is painful for some people and can cause potential damage to the lining of the esophagus.

Smoking can lead to other serious health problems, including cancer. The chemicals found in cigarettes are considered carcinogenic. This means that the more you are exposed to cigarette and its smoke, the more predisposed you are to developing cancer. If no immediate action is taken to stop smoking, irreversible damages can happen and death may be unavoidable. In contrast, quitting smoking as early as possible, can contribute to a higher life expectancy.

If you are unsure where to start, here are essential tips you can use in smoking cessation:

- Quitting smoking is not an overnight process. You have to take the process of weaning seriously.

- Set a specific date when you'll stop smoking and follow it.

- Avoid keeping cigarettes at home or anywhere with you.

- Keep yourself away from situations or events where you'd normally smoke.

- Practice delay. Avoid giving in right away if you are tempted to smoke.

- Find a good distraction. You can chew on something else, such as a sugarless gum or a hard candy.

- Consider nicotine replacement therapy if you can't handle the urge to smoke.

Chapter 7

Exercise Your Way to a Healthy Gut

Apparently, food types and supplements aren't the only ones that can trigger various microbe formations in your gut. Exercise can also do that for you. In a collaborative study conducted by the University College of Cork and the National University of Ireland, exercise has a direct effect on the diversity of bacteria in the gut. A separate study was also able to point out the ability of exercise to reverse gut flora associated with obesity.

Exercise, in general, is helpful for your gut. Being physically active, even though it's as simple as a daily walk, can aid in better digestion. It also helps you achieve stronger abdominal muscles and eliminate the possibility of gaining too much weight. Exercising for your gut health can be as light or as difficult as you can. Ideally, you need to dedicate around thirty minutes each day to be physically active. If your work or daily chores don't permit you to exercise, you can try to choose actions that will physically benefit you and incorporate them in your daily activities. Walking to the parking area or using the stairs is simple yet effective in keeping you moving and active.

However, not all exercises are fit for everyone. As such, you should still be careful in selecting your type of exercise. Forcing your body to do an exercise beyond your capacity can cause toxins from your gut to leak out and enter your systemic circulation. When this happens, a systemic immune response can happen. Instead of making you healthier, it can actually be more harmful for your health.

Chapter 8

The Role of Probiotics

Probiotics refer to the good bacteria or organisms that provide a multitude of health benefits. Most commonly, they can be found in fermented foods such as yogurt and kefir. Today, however, probiotics aren't limited to foods. As a matter of fact, you can easily purchase them in form of supplements and they are fairly increasing in number.

There are various strains of probiotics. The most common strains you'll encounter are the lactobacillus and bifidobacterium. The lactobacillus strain is mostly found in milk and fermented products. These probiotics are helpful for people with diarrhea and those who are intolerant to lactose. One of the most known strains of lactobacillus is the Lactobacillus Acidophilus. It helps make nutrient absorption easier by colonizing the lining of the small intestine.

Bifidobacterium, on the other hand, is also present in several dairy products. Inside your gut, this strain is more populated in small and large intestine. They are beneficial for people suffering from Irritable Bowel Syndrome. The most popular strain from bifidobacterium is the B. Bifidum. These probiotics help in breaking down carbohydrates, protein and fats into forms which can easily be processed and assimilated by the body.

Probiotics play a big role in your gut health, particularly in the normal flora of your digestive track. These microorganisms help maintain the balance of the good and bad bacteria in your system. They prevent the bad ones from proliferating and causing trouble in your gut. In one study, published by the Journal of Pediatrics, probiotics, when used as prophylaxis, can help reduce the chances of nosocomial diarrhea from happening to infants. They are also established to be effective in preventing or treating several disorders of the gastrointestinal track.

Aside from disease prevention, probiotics can also help improve your digestion and aid in your weight loss. They have also been known to be effective in enhancing one's immunity, managing depression, and in normalizing cholesterol and blood pressure level.

There are several sources of probiotics in the market. Most of them can easily be found in your own kitchen.

This includes yogurt, miso, and even kimchi. If you are not fond of these food types, you can easily purchase probiotic supplements today. However, you should take note that, unlike prescription medicines, supplements are not strictly regulated. To find the best probiotic supplement, you should consider examining what strains of probiotics are included, the expiration date of the supplement and how it can get to you. Time and processing are important factors to consider, especially if you want to make sure you get good, healthy and live microorganisms for your gut.

Chapter 9

De-stress for a Healthier Digestion

It's normal for a person to feel stressed out from time to time. However, being exposed to stress for a long period of time can take a toll on your health, particularly your gut. This happens with the activation of the body's "fight or flight' response during stress. During this process, the central nervous system gets triggered and the digestive system gets shut down to give way for more blood to enter the main circulation. With decreased blood flow to your gut, several harmful effects occur.

Stress can decrease the production of enzymes in your gut. These enzymes are essential in the digestion of food and absorption of nutrients. A decrease in enzyme means there'll be a decline in the amount of nutrients your body receives. Stress can also lead to excessive acid production. When this happens, the lining of your gut can easily get irritated and damaged. Constipation, irritable bowel syndrome and stomach ulcers, then, becomes inevitable.

By knowing how stress can affect your gut health, you'll also have a good idea on how you can combat it. Actually, there are a lot of de-stressing techniques you can do to minimize the impact of stress on your digestive health. Here are some of them:

Practice relaxation techniques. Yoga, meditation and deep breathing techniques are some of the most common ways to eliminate stress. These techniques are easy to learn and do on your own. However, for more advanced techniques like hypnosis and biofeedback, you can seek the help of professional therapists.

Take enough rest. Sleep allows your body to relax and repair itself. Without the right amount of sleep every night, you're likely to get weak in resisting stress and its debilitating effects. For optimum health, you can try to get at least 6 hours of sleep.

Go out. Exploring nature can also be a good way of relieving stress. Taking time to walk alone in the park or simply take a minute to breath fresh air can help calm your mind. Socialization is also helpful. Being with friends and enjoying group activities are good stress relievers.

Express yourself. Containing stress and emotions isn't helpful. As a matter of fact, it can only make matters worse. There are several ways for you to unload. Talking to your friends, for one, can help you get things off of your chest. Keeping a daily journal can also aid you in expressing frustrations and other emotions. If these methods aren't helpful, there are trained therapists who can assist you in coping better with chronic stress.

Chapter 10

How to Handle Food Allergies

Food allergies can be debilitating. It can cause great discomfort, pain and even embarrassment. Some cases are excessively limiting in that a person never gets to eat a certain food for most of his life. On severe cases, food allergies trigger an anaphylactic reaction. This involves swelling of the lips and mouth, tightening of the airway, and wheezing. Weakening of the pulse, chest pain and shortness of breath are also fairly common. If no immediate action is taken, it can lead to potentially lethal life threats.

Food allergies are very common. In fact, its frequency doubles because of cross reactivity. A person, for example, who is allergic to a shellfish, can also be allergic to shrimps and other sea foods. Because of this, achieving definitive diagnosis can be difficult. You'll need to consult with an immunologist or an allergist to make sure all possible allergens are considered and tested.

A healthy gut, however, can give you protection against most food allergies. This is reflected in a study released by experts from University of Chicago Medicine and Biological Studies. The research was able to find out that a certain type of probiotic, specifically Clostridia, can help reduce the allergen level in the blood.

Leaking Gut Syndrome, on the other hand, is also considered as a major factor on why food allergies happen. Because the barrier in the gut is hyper permeable, a lot of substance in the digestive track can leak and trigger several immune reactions in the body. Aside from food allergies and intolerances, Leaking Gut Syndrome can also trigger bloating, diarrhea, hormonal imbalances and even autoimmune diseases.

In managing food allergies, your primary objective is to remove all possible allergens and triggers. This can include inflammatory foods and possible infections. Once you have gotten rid of these factors, you can start replacing the nutrients and ingredients your gut needs in order to be healthy. Special diets can also be considered in managing food allergies. Most of the time, it's actually the single most effective way in handling food intolerances.

However, because technology is a lot more advanced today, treatment approaches, such as immunotherapy, are becoming more common. Immunotherapy involves altering a person's immune response to an allergen. A patient undergoes provocation and neutralization of his allergy until the right "neutralizing dose" is attained. He can inject the solution by himself or take it by mouth in case he consumes an allergenic food.

Chapter 11

How to Prepare a Diet Plan

So, now that you have learned what makes up a Gut Balance Diet and the tons of advantages you can obtain from including it in your day-to-day life, the next question is -- how can I start preparing my Gut Balance diet plan?

Many first-timers tend to get overwhelmed by the idea. Most people have the false impression that getting into the Gut Balance Diet would be too limiting or restricting.

Well, here's the good news – there are tons of possibilities and you can find yourself swimming in a sea of recipes. There are way too many options. On the plus side, you also have the option to reinvent your loved recipes but simply replacing some of the ingredients. And if you happen to be taking some baby steps, here are important tips to guide you all you way to a healthier version of yourself:

TIP #01: You can eat the amount that you NEED

Please note the word 'NEED' and not 'WANT'. Gut healing and strengthening also requires eating the right quantity that your body needs. There is a recommended 'serving size' for every meal. However, it is up to you to make a certain adjustment based on all your adjacent activities. To put simply, you can increase the quantity of your food if you work out often. The more you exercise, the more you can eat. Moreover, you can eat until you are 80% full. Again, you do not need to be stuffed to be nourished. Being 80% is better for your digestive health, gut balance, nutrition absorption, and yes, metabolism.

TIP #02: Know how you can support yourself effectively

As the Gut Balance Diet is primary to promote gut healing, you can expect diet plans packed with low-in-sugar components. Carbohydrates are also kept to a minimum. This could particularly be difficult for people who are quite dependent on carbohydrate for energy. To supplement your diet, you can include complex carbohydrates to meet you energy needs. Top choices for Gut Balance are peas, lentils, quinoa, and root crops. Adding a dash of protein powder or some extra fats to your smoothies can be particularly helpful, too.

TIP #03: You can add a bit of your personality to your food

Healthy food does not have to be bland - AT ALL! You can personalize your food by loading more veggies, choosing healthier types of fats and including protein to your meal. This can make your gut-friendly dish tastier and more palatable. The trick is to understand what must and must NOT go to your plate. Note that the Gut Balance Diet is to ensure that you have a clean gut all the time – so as to promote health and better digestion. If you would like to have a quick recap on the basic food Dos and Don'ts, then feel free to see the list below:

Say BONJOUR to these foods

- Loads of fresh vegetables

- Go gaga over Greens

- Wild Fish

- Berries   (either fresh or frozen)

- A small serving a day of quinoa

- A handful of nuts or seeds

- More lentils

- Never forego of avocados

- Fermented side dishes (sauerkraut, kimchi)

- Olive oil

- Coconut oil

- Meats that are grass-fed ONLY

- Organic eggs

Say ADIEU to these foods

- Dairy

- Gluten

- Alcohol

- Caffeine-laden food and drinks

- Potatoes

- Soy

- Corn

- Beans

- Rice

- Almost all types of fruit

- Processed sugar

Chapter 12: Your 4-Week Gut Balance Diet Plan

If planning you meals can be a bit tedious, then you can follow the 4-week plan provided below. The concept is to provide you with an option to get help you reboot and renew your entire gut and digestive system. As stated in the previous chapter, you can also give this diet plan your personal touch as long as you take note of the quantity as well as the components you include in the dish.

Week 1	Day 1	Day 2	Day 3	Day 4	Day 5	Day 6	Day 7
Breakfast	Vanilla and Almond Shake	Green Coconut Shake	Chocolate Ginger smoothie	Coco-Chai Shake	Clean Choco Drink	Mint Chip Shake	Fruit-free all-green smoothie
Snack	Celery Sticks with Almond Butter	Carrot sticks with Strawberry Ginger Dressing	Roasted Broccoli with Tahini Dip	Crackers with Guacamole	Hard-boiled eggs	A handful of mixed nuts	Gluten-free crackers with sunflower seed pate
Lunch	Coconut Crusted Haddock	Vegetable Chili and Quinoa	Buffalo Cauliflower in Cashew Ranch Dressing	Turkey Meatballs in Tomato Dijon	Crockpot Turkey Breast	Beef with Parsley, Lemon, and Onion	Chicken Thighs Pesto
Snack	Zucchini Humus	Wheat Crackers and Artichoke Dip	Sunflower seed pate and rice-free crackers	Pumpkin seed pesto	Vegetable medley with Avocado dip	One large banana	Celery and Humus
Dinner	Salmon Chowder	Creamy Pumpkin Soup	Lettuce in coconut soup	Mushroom Soup with Cauliflower	Kale Soup with Turkey Sausage	Acorn Squash Soup	Dairy-free Creamy Asparagus Soup
Treat	Aloe Vera Jelly Cubes	Clean Gut Pudding Pie	Protein Cheesecake	Mini Red velvet cupcakes	Ginger Apple crisp	Mocha and Banana Ice cream (dairy-free)	Clean Chocolate Brownie

Week 2	Day 1	Day 2	Day 3	Day 4	Day 5	Day 6	Day 7
Breakfast	Spiced Raspberry Shake	Avocado and Hemp Seed Shake	Fruit-free all-green smoothie	Blueberry Almond Shake	Euro Nutty Shake	Chocolate Covered Blueberries	Superwoman's all-green shake
Snack	Basil and Pesto Hummus	Balsamic Bruschetta	Crackers and Lentil Dip	Granola Bar	A handful of mixed nuts	Celery with Hummus	Carrot sticks with Strawberry Ginger Dressing
Lunch	Chicken Pot Pie	Turkey Meatballs in Tomato Dijon	Salmon and Asparagus Parchment	Garam Masala Chicken	Beef with Parsley, Lemon, and Onion	Chicken and Waffles	Chicken Nuggets with Thai Dip
Snack	Balsamic Bruschetta	Celery and Avocado Salsa	Artichokes with Mustard and Lemon Dip	Roasted Eggplant with Garlic Hummus	Cinnamon Vanilla Granola	Celery and Humus	Vegetable medley with Avocado dip
Dinner	Crockpot Turkey Breast	Mushroom Soup with Cauliflower	Salmon Chowder	Roasted Broccoli Soup	Roasted Winter Squash with lentils	Ginger Lemon Stir Fry	Dairy-free Creamy Asparagus Soup
Treat	Almond milk with Stevia	Malted Maca Milkshake	Mocha and Banana Ice cream (dairy-free)	Coco Raspberry Popsicle	Gluten-free and flour-free chocolate brownie	Turmeric Latte with Honey	Ginger Apple crisp

Week 3	Day 1	Day 2	Day 3	Day 4	Day 5	Day 6	Day 7
Breakfast	Fruit-free all-green smoothie	Blueberry Cinnamon Shake	Purple Mason Jar Shake	Grasshopper Shake	Avocado and Spinach Shake	Mint Chip Shake	Chocolate Ginger smoothie
Snack	Baked Kale Chips	Spiced Sweet Roasted Pepper with Hummus	Cinnamon Vanilla Granola	Crackers with Guacamole	Gluten-free crackers with sunflower seed pate	Balsamic Bruschetta	Tofu Hummus
Lunch	Spinach and Chard Souffle	Vegetable Frittata	Chicken Thighs Pesto	Beef with Parsley, Lemon, and Onion	Zucchini Spaghetti	Parchment Halibut and Olives	Roasted Winter Squash with lentils
Snack	Crackers with Cucumber Hummus	Balsamic Bruschetta	Vegetable medley with Avocado dip	Celery and Humus	Artichokes with Mustard and Lemon Dip	Lentil Pate	Spiced granola bar
Dinner	Mediterranean Bean Salad	Mushroom Soup	Chicken Nuggets with Thai Dip	Parchment Halibut and Olives	Salmon and Asparagus Parchment	Spring Chicken and Vegetable Soup	Gingered Squash Soup
Treat	Herbal Tea with Stevia and honey	Mocha and Banana Ice cream (dairy-free)	Gluten-free and flour-free chocolate brownie	Ginger Apple crisp	Coco Raspberry Popsicle	Almond milk with Stevia	Turmeric Latte with Honey

Week 4	Day 1	Day 2	Day 3	Day 4	Day 5	Day 6	Day 7
Breakfast	Spiced Raspberry Shake	Vanilla Nutty Shake	Chocolate Ginger smoothie	Aloe Vera Shake	All Favorite Shake	Superwoman's all-green shake	Avocado and Hemp Seed Shake
Snack	Spiced Sweet Roasted Pepper with Hummus	Celery Sticks with Almond Butter	Balsamic Bruschetta	A handful of mixed nuts	Lentil Pate	Crackers with Cucumber Hummus	Spiced granola bar
Lunch	Roasted Winter Squash with lentils	Chicken Pot Pie	Vegetable Chili and Quinoa	Deconstructed California Maki	Braised Beef and Mashed Cauliflower	Herb Chicken Verde	Vegetable Frittata
Snack	Roasted Eggplant with Garlic Hummus	Almond milk with Stevia	Vegetable medley with Avocado dip	Tofu Hummus	Baked Kale Chips	Carrot sticks with Strawberry Ginger Dressing	Balsamic Bruschetta
Dinner	Summer vegetable Kelp Noodles	Salmon and Asparagus Parchment	Roasted Broccoli Soup	Mushroom Soup with Cauliflower	Vegetable Barley Soup	Chicken Nuggets with Thai Dip	Creamy Pumpkin Soup
Treat	Hazel Nut Coco crunch Bar	Gluten-free and flour-free chocolate brownie	Protein Cheesecake	Almond milk with Stevia	Malted Maca Milkshake	Aloe Vera Jelly Cubes	Coco Raspberry Popsicle

Bonus Chapter

Recipes You Can Follow

OK, Let's start with the endless varieties of Gut Balance Morning Shakes to help you obtain the right energy you need in the morning while maintaining a healthy and clean gut.

BREAKFAST GUT-BALANCE SHAKES

Fruit Free All- Green Smoothie

Inspired by Sonnet's Kitchen

½ organic cucumber, roughly chopped

½ avocado, peeled

2 cups organic spinach

¼ cup chopped parsley

½ lemon, peeled

1 cup coconut water

6-10 cubes

Blend all ingredients together until smooth.

Blueberry Cinnamon Shake

1 cup almond milk

½ cup of frozen blueberries or raspberries

1 tablespoon of organic raw coconut butter

1 tablespoon of Clean Greens

1 cinnamon stick

1 packet protein powder

 1 tablespoon ground flax seed

Blend all ingredients together until smooth.

Chocolate Ginger Shake

1 cup of unsweetened choco almond milk

1" ginger, peeled and grated or finely chopped

1 heaping tablespoon cacao or cocoa powder

1 heaping tablespoon cashew or sunflower seed butter

Add stevia to taste

1 packet protein powder

Blend until smooth and creamy.

Avocado Hempseed Shake

8 ounces of water

½ of an avocado

3-4 ounces of unsweetened hemp seed

2 teaspoons organic almond butter

A pinch of sea salt

1 packet protein powder

tablespoon ground flax seed

Blend until smooth

*replace hempseed with spinach to make it for another morning shake recipe

Coco Chai Shake

1 cup coconut milk (unsweetened)

1 tablespoon vanilla extract

1 teaspoon ginger

1 teaspoon cinnamon

¼ cup shredded coconut

A pinch of allspice

2 tablespoons almond or cashew butter

1 packet protein powder

tablespoon ground flax seed

Blend until smooth and creamy.

Spiced Raspberry shake

2 cups fresh almond milk

1 cup frozen raspberries

1 teaspoon cinnamon

¼ teaspoon freshly grated nutmeg

¼ teaspoon stevia

Pinch of sea salt

1 packet protein powder

Blend until smooth and creamy.

Chocolate Covered Blueberries

1 large handful of frozen or fresh blueberries

1 handful of spinach

Dash of cinnamon

1 tablespoon of raw cacao

2 tablespoons almond butter

½ coconut milk and ½ coconut water

Dash of stevia as needed

1 packet protein powder add tablespoon ground flax seed

Blend until creamy.

** You may add green tea for added flavor

Euro Nutty Shake

1 cup unsweetened coconut milk

1 tablespoon vanilla extract

Stevia to taste

2 tablespoons raw cacao

2-4 tablespoons hazelnut butter

6-10 ice cubes1 packet protein powder

add 1 tablespoon ground flax seed

Blend until creamy!

Green Shake

3 cups spinach

1 tablespoon flax oil

1 tablespoon maca powder

1 tablespoon spirulina

1 cup almond milk

A few drops of stevia t

1 packet protein powder

Blend until creamy.

Morning Mocha Shake

1 cup strong teeccino

2 tablespoons cacao powder

1 handful of raw almonds

1 tablespoon vanilla extract

1 packet protein powder (choco-flavored)

add 1 tablespoon ground flax seed

Stevia to taste

Blend until creamy.

Aloe Vera Shake

From the Clean Team

1 large aloe vera gel (you may also get aloe vera leaves and scrape off the flesh)

1 cup coconut water

Juice of 1 lemon

1 cup organic berries

2 handfuls of spinach, kale, chard, or any mix of organic greens

Add Stevia to taste

1 packet protein powder

Blend all ingredients but add aloe vera gel in the end

All Favorite Shake

Frozen blueberries

1 cup Lacinato kale

Unsweetened almond milk

1 tablespoon almond butter

1 packet protein shake

add 1 tablespoon ground flax seed

Blend until smooth.

Blueberry Almond Shake

1 cup almond milk

½ cup of frozen blueberries

½ cup matcha green tea

1 tablespoon of organic raw coconut butter

1 packet protein powder (choco-flavored)

add 1 tablespoon ground flax seed

Blend until creamy.

Blueberry Cinnamon Shake

½ cup frozen blueberries

2 dashes cinnamon

1 tablespoon almond butter

8 ounces of water

1 packet Clean Shakes Chocolate (or other protein powder)

Optional: 1 tablespoon ground flax seed

Add 6-10 ice cubes

Blend until creamy.

Vanilla Almond Shake

2 cups almond milk (fresh would be better)

1 tablespoon vanilla extract

1 heaping tablespoon almond butter

1 teaspoon cinnamon

½ teaspoon nutmeg

A dash of sea salt

dash of stevia to taste

1 packet protein powder

Blend until smooth.

Green Superwoman Shake

Adapted from Healthful Pursuit

1 cup unsweetened almond milk

1 cup spinach

1 tablespoon cacao powder

1 tablespoon almond butter

1 tablespoon coconut oil

Stevia to taste

1 teaspoon spirulina

1 cup frozen mixed berries

6-10 ice cubes

1 packet protein powder

add tablespoon ground flax seed

Blend until creamy.

Grasshopper Shake

1 heaping tablespoon cacao powder

2 teaspoons spirulina

1½ cups warm peppermint tea

2 tablespoon whole cashews

Pinch of sea salt

¼ teaspoon stevia

1 packet powder shake

add tablespoon ground flax seed

Blend everything and warm. Serve as a warm drink.

Purple Mason Jar Shake

1 cup almond milk, unsweetened

½ cup fresh or frozen organic blueberries

1 tablespoon spirulina

2 tablespoons almond butter

1 tablespoon tahini

1 teaspoon vanilla

Add a few drops of stevia

1 packet protein powder

Blend until Smooth

Green Coco Shake

2 cups coconut water

1 handful baby spinach

1 ripe avocado, pitted

3 tablespoons whole cashews

Pinch of stevia

1 packet protein powder

Blend until smooth

Vanilla Nut Shake

1 cup almond milk

2 heaping tablespoons nut butter (almond or pecan)

1/2 cup water

Pinch of sea salt

2 teaspoons vanilla (pure powder or extract)

1 tablespoon maca

Stevia to taste

Blend until smooth.

Green Tea Shake

Warm green tea

2 tablespoons coconut oil

¼ avocado

A couple dashes cinnamon

A few drops of

1 packet protein powder

add 1 tablespoon ground flax seed

add 6-10 ice cubes

Blend until creamy.

Avocado and Spinach Shake

1 cup fresh blueberries

1 cup fresh spinach leaves

1 cup almond milk

½ ripe avocado

1 tablespoon chia seeds

¼ teaspoon cinnamon

Stevia to taste

1 packet protein powder

½ cup fresh ice

Blend until smooth

FOR SNACKS AND SALADS, YOU CAN TRY THESE GUT-BALANCE DRESSINGS AND DIPS

Avocado Dressing

2 ripe avocados, chopped

2 spring onions, finely chopped

1 clove garlic, minced

2 tablespoons lime juice

½ teaspoon cider vinegar

Water to think

Sea salt, to taste

Whisk well and enjoy!

Best Balsamic Dressing

3 cloves garlic minced

1 tablespoon mustard

1 tablespoon gluten-free miso

¼ cup balsamic vinegar

2 tablespoons wheat-free tamari

½ cup olive oil

Salt and pepper to taste

Whisk until well-blended

Gut-Balance Caesar Dressing

1 cup raw cashews (soaked for 4 hours)

Juice of 1 lemon

3 cloves garlic minced

¼ cup nutritional yeast

3 tablespoons wheat-free tamari

1 tablespoon gluten-free miso

3 tablespoons extra virgin olive oil

1 tablespoon Dijon mustard

Anchovy fillets (3-5 pieces)

salt and pepper to taste

Use water to think.

Ginger Dressing

½ cup olive oil

½ cup water

2 teaspoons ground ginger

2 tablespoons red wine vinegar

¼ cup wheat-free tamari

2 tablespoons lemon juice

1 garlic clove, finely minced

Black pepper and salt to taste

Whisk well. Store in fridge, but consume within 72 hours.

Guacamole Dip

2 avocados

1 clove garlic, peeled and minced

1/4 of a red onion, peeled and finely diced

Zest of a lemon or lime

Juice of 1 lime

Finely chopped cilantro

Sea salt

Mash all ingredients together in a bowl to desired consistency. Serve with gluten free crackers or vegetables.

Zucchini Hummus

4 cups zucchini

¾ cup sesame tahini

Juice of 4 lemons

¼ cup olive oil

4 garlic cloves

1 tablespoon cumin

2 teaspoons sea salt

¼ teaspoon paprika

Plug in your blender or food processor, place all ingredients (except for the paprika)

And blend away. You can replace Zucchini with other vegetables to make hummus. Add paprika before serving. Serve with gluten free crackers or vegetables.

Sunflower Seed Pate

2 1/2 cups sunflower seeds which have been soaked for 2 whole hours

1/4 cup sauerkraut or kimchi

2 celery sticks, roughly chopped

1/4 cup shallot

Juice of 1 lemon

1/4 cup olive oil

1/4 cup freshly chopped herbs (rosemary and thyme)

Sea salt to taste.

Use veggies such as cucumber, celery, peppers, etc for serving

Chop the ingredients to make the texture consistent. Then blend all of them using a food processor until you have your desired consistency.

Use as salad topping or for noodles. This can be eaten with crackers and vegetables too.

For LUNCH AND DINNER, here are our TOP 8 choices:

Chicken Nuggets with Thai Dipping Sauce

For the Chicken Nuggets:

2 tablespoons almond milk (unsweetened)

1 cup almond meal

1 egg

1 teaspoon garlic powder

1 teaspoon sea salt

1 tablespoon apple cider vinegar

1 teaspoon chili powder

¼ cup olive oil

5 cloves garlic, peeled and minced

1 tablespoon freshly ground pepper

1 large or 2 small boneless chicken breasts

Chopped parsley for garnishing

For the Thai Sauce:

1 1/2 cups dry-roasted almond butter

1 teaspoons red chili paste

1/4 cup glutton-free miso paste

1 tablespoon minced fresh ginger root or 2 teaspoons ginger powder

Add 1 or two drops stevia

Juice of 1 lime

1/4 cup coconut milk

** add all these and blend until you arrive at a creamy consistency

Preheat oven to 425 ⁰ F and line a baking sheet with parchment paper. Prepare the chicken coating. In a small bowl, whisk together the egg and non-dairy milk. In another bowl, add garlic, almond oatmeal, and salt. Dip the chicken in the egg and milk mixture then coat it with the almond oatmeal and garlic mixture. Drizzle with olive oil and bake for 8 minutes. Serve with the Thai sauce and some greens.

Summer Vegetable Kelp Noodles

1 large summer squash cut into quarters

2 tablespoons olive oil

2 handful of shitake mushroom

1 bulb of fennel

4 garlic cloves, thinly sliced

¼ cup pine nuts

2 tablespoons fresh chopped basil or rosemary

1 package kelp noodles

Remove the kelp noodles as prepare as per package instructions. Slice the squash, fennel, and shitake mushrooms. Heat a saucepan over medium-high heat then add the olive oil and the sliced garlic. Toss in the squash, fennel, and shitake mushrooms. Using a wooden spoon, continuously stir so as to prevent the garlic from burning. Add the kelp noodles and stir for a few more minutes. Add the basil and season it with a bit of salt.   Garnish with pine nuts. Serve warm and enjoy.

Spaghetti Squash with Cauliflower Sauce

For the spaghetti squash

1 spaghetti squash

1 - 2 teaspoons organic extra virgin olive oil

1 large organic red bell pepper

1/4 cup organic fresh basil, chopped

1 cup shitake mushroom diced

1 small organic onion, chopped

2 tablespoons organic coconut oil

For the cauliflower sauce:

1 large organic cauliflower

2 cups fresh almond milk

5 cloves organic garlic, crushed and finely minced

2 tablespoons nutritional yeast

Pink Himalayan salt

1 pinches organic cayenne pepper

Prepare the spaghetti squash pasta by cutting it and removing the seed. Rub a generous amount of olive oil on the inside of the spaghetti squash and bake it for 45 minutes. Prepare the sauce by boiling the cauliflower for 15 minutes. Blend it with the rest of the ingredients until creamy. Prepare vegetables by sauteing the red bell peppers and onions. Toss the mushroom and cook until tender. Combine all sautéed vegetables and the sauce and top them onto the pasta. Garnish with fresh basil when serving.

Parchment Halibut with Olives

1 large halibut piece (this is good for 2 servings)

1 fennel bulb

2 parsnips

Cold pressed olive oil

Lemon of 1 juice

1/3 cup mixed olives (green, black, kalamata)

Parchment paper

Peel and chop the parsnips while boiling water in a medium pot. Place the parsnips in the water when it's at boiling point and let it cook for 8 minutes. Check if parsnips are tender with a fork.

Slice the fennel bulb. Make sure you remove the stems and the outer skin. Slice the lemon into thin rounds. In a large bowl combine the piece of halibut with the lemon slices, fennel pieces, fennel fronds and the olives. Drain the cooked parsnips and add them in the halibut mixture. Drizzle the mixture with some oil (1-2 tablespoons).

Ensure that everything is well coated. Place everything onto the center of a large piece of parchment paper. Add all remaining juices on top of the halibut to keep it moist. Fold up the edges of the bag and seal the edges. Put the parchment halibut in a baking pan. Preheat the oven to 400 º F and place the halibut in. Cook the package for 20-25 minutes depending on the thickness of the fish. Remove from oven when the parchment color turns golden brown. Open the parchment and serve warm.

Thai Coconut Chicken Soup

A few spoonfuls of coconut oil

2 cans coconut milk

½ red onion, chopped

2 garlic cloves, minced

1 jalapeño seeded and chopped

4 cups vegetable or chicken broth

2 inch grated ginger

1 cup of mushrooms chopped

Zest and juice of 1 lemon or lime

3-4 tablespoons fish sauce

2 stalks lemongrass

1 pound chicken sliced thinly

8 cherry tomatoes

Fresh cilantro chopped for garnish

A dash of Wheat-free tamari

Dash of stevia

Melt coconut oil in a soup pot. Add jalapeño, onions and garlic and saute for 2 minutes. Slowly incorporate the coconut milk, broth, ginger, lemongrass, fish sauce, and chicken to the soup pot. Add the lime zest. Let it simmer for 12-15 minutes. Toss in the mushrooms, tomato, dash of stevia and lime juice to the pot. Simmer for another 5 minutes. Garnish with cilantro.

Gingered Salmon Stir Fry

8 ounces of wild salmon (fillet) and cut into desired sizes

1 carrot cut into thin rounds

1 cup snow peas sliced into thin pieces

2 tablespoons sesame oil

1 bunch scallions diced

2 tablespoons grated ginger

1 garlic clove, peeled and minced

1/4 cup dry roasted cashews

organic brown rice vinegar

Season the salmon pieces with sea salt and black pepper. Heat a large saute pan over high heat then add sesame oil. Add the salmon pieces and brown each side for 2 minutes. Add the vegetable and continuously toss. Add the garlic and the ginger. When the fragrance starts to burst, add a dash of brown rice vinegar. Place the lid on and simmer for 2 minutes. Add the scallions and cashews and let cook for 30 seconds. Serve warm.

Coriander Crusted Halibut

2 halibut fillets

½ kg of carrots

2 tablespoons of coarsely ground coriander seed

A generous amount of olive oil

A tablespoon of sea salt

Fresh ground pepper

2 tablespoons coconut oil

For the Parsley Sauce:

½ bunch of parsley (make sure you remove the stalks)

1 garlic clove, finely chopped

Juice and zest of 1 lemon

½ cup of olive oil

Preheat oven to 375 º F. Prepare the vegetables first. Toss the carrots and splash with salt, olive oil, and a fresh ground black pepper. Bake until lightly brown. Check if tender by using a fork. Remove from oven and set aside. Start grinding coriander seed until course in texture. Sprinkle some on the surface of the fish fillet. Heat a pan with coconut oil and sear the fish on each side for 3-4 minutes. Do not overcook as this could turn the fish dry. For the parsley sauce, puree all the ingredients. Place carrots on a plate and put the fish on top of it. Drizzle with Parsley sauce.

Summer Squash and Tomato Bake

2-3 large summer squash into ¼ inch thick pieces

3 garlic cloves, minced

3 medium sized shallots

2-3 tablespoons coconut oil

1-quart tomato puree

3 anchovies, (you can add more depending on your personal taste)

2 tablespoons capers, minced

½ cup chopped green olives

¼ cup parsley, finely chopped

¼ cup basil, torn into smaller pieces

Sea salt and pepper to taste

**Add protein such as chicken breast, turkey, or lentils

Preheat the oven to 350 º F. Saute sliced shallots using 3-4 tablespoons of coconut or vegetable oil. Add the garlic when shallots turned translucent. Add the anchovies, olives, and the capers for about 2-3 minutes then pour the quarter cup tomato puree. Simmer for 15 minutes under low heat.

In another sauce pan, spoon and spread a layer of the sauce. Then, spread the sliced squash onto the sauce and top again with more sauce. Add pepper and salt to taste. Continue working on the layers and then place in the oven and bake for half an hour.

Conclusion

The gut is probably one of the most underappreciated systems in the human body. It's also one of the most overlooked causes of the multitude of health issues we are experiencing today. Because of the recent advancements in technology and medicine, however, the close relationship between the gastrointestinal system and the overall human health is slowly being established. Little by little, we're starting to learn more about it.

Taking care of your gut isn't really as hard as you think. As a matter of fact, you only need to be more considerate and attentive to what your system is actually telling you. By taking time to listen to your gut, you'll be able to understand your body better. After all, there is such a thing as "gut feeling" and it's almost always right.

Printed in Great Britain
by Amazon